WATER AEROBICS FOR SENIORS

COPYRIGHT

All rights reserved

TABLE OF CONTENTS

3. Toe Touches

Cardiovascular Exercises

Water Walking

Jogging in Place

Kickboarding

Strength and Resistance Exercises

Leg Lifts

Arm Curls

Water Dumbbell Exercises

knee excercises

arthritis excercises

hip excercises

shoulder excercises

back and waist excercises

Flexibility and Stretching Exercises

Side Stretches

Chest Opener

1

INTRODUCTION TO WATER AEROBICS FOR SENIORS

Water aerobics is a low-impact form of exercise that is ideal for seniors who want to stay active and improve their physical fitness. It offers a multitude of health benefits while being gentle on the joints, making it a popular choice among older adults.

Water aerobics is typically conducted in a shallow pool, allowing participants to exercise while buoyant in the water. This reduces the strain on joints and muscles, minimizing the risks of injury. Seniors with arthritis or other joint conditions often find relief in water aerobics, as the water provides a natural resistance that helps to strengthen muscles without putting excessive pressure on the joints.

One of the main advantages of water aerobics for seniors is its cardiovascular benefits. It increases heart rate and improves circulation, which in turn contributes to a healthier heart and lowers the risk of cardiovascular diseases. Regular water aerobics can also help to manage blood pressure and reduce cholesterol levels.

In addition, water aerobics is an effective way to improve balance and coordination, which are crucial for reducing the risk of falls in older adults. The supportive nature of water helps to build strength in the core muscles, improving stability in seniors. This is especially important as falls can lead to serious injuries and fractures, making water aerobics a valuable activity for fall prevention.

Water aerobics can have positive effects on mental health as well. The serene environment of the pool, combined with the social interaction among participants, can help combat feelings of loneliness and isolation commonly experienced by seniors. Regular exercise in water has also been shown to reduce symptoms of anxiety and depression, promoting overall well-being.

Water aerobics is an excellent form of exercise for seniors to improve their physical and mental health. Its low-impact nature, cardiovascular benefits, improvement of balance and coordination, and positive effects on mental well-being make it an ideal activity for older adults. Whether you are a senior looking for an enjoyable way to stay fit or a caregiver seeking a suitable exercise option, water aerobics is worth exploring for all the potential advantages it offers.

BENEFITS OF WATER AEROBICS FOR SENIORS

Water aerobics, has gained popularity among seniors due to its numerous benefits for overall health and fitness. This low-impact form of exercise is particularly beneficial for seniors as it helps improve their cardiovascular health, flexibility, strength, and balance.

One of the main advantages of water aerobics for seniors is its low-impact nature. The buoyancy of water reduces the impact on joints, making it an ideal exercise for individuals with arthritis or joint problems. It provides a gentle way to stay active and maintain mobility without putting excessive strain on the body.

Water aerobics also improves cardiovascular health. The resistance provided by water increases the heart rate, helping to strengthen the heart and improve circulation. Regular participation in water aerobics can decrease the risk of cardiovascular diseases such as high blood pressure, heart disease, and stroke.

Furthermore, water aerobics helps enhance flexibility and range of motion. The water's resistance allows for a wide range of movements, stretching and toning muscles in a gentle manner. This is particularly beneficial for seniors as it can help alleviate stiffness and improve joint flexibility.

Strength and balance are also areas where seniors can benefit from water aerobics. Water provides natural resistance, making each movement more challenging and assisting in building muscle strength. Additionally, the buoyancy of water helps support the body, providing a safe environment for balance exercises.

Water aerobics sessions are often conducted in groups, which provides an opportunity for social interaction and the chance to meet new people. This social aspect helps to reduce feelings of isolation and can improve mental well-being.

Water aerobics offers a multitude of benefits for seniors. Its low-impact nature, ability to improve cardiovascular health, flexibility, strength, and balance, makes it an ideal exercise option for seniors to stay fit and active. So, grab your swimsuit, and join a water aerobics class to experience the positive impact on your overall health and well-being.

HOW WATER AEROBICS CAN IMPROVE HEALTH AND FITNESS

This form of exercise is suitable for people of all ages and fitness levels. Water aerobics can help individuals improve their cardiovascular health, muscular strength, flexibility, and overall physical fitness.

One significant advantage of water aerobics is the reduced impact on joints and bones. The buoyancy of water reduces the stress on the body, making it an excellent exercise option for individuals with joint pain, arthritis, or other musculoskeletal conditions. Compared to traditional aerobics, water aerobics puts less strain on the knees, hips, and back, while offering similar cardiovascular benefits.

Additionally, water resistance provides an added challenge to the muscles, leading to increased muscle strength and endurance. The resistance of water is about twelve times greater than air, making movements in the water more challenging than on land. By performing exercises like water jogging, leg lifts, arm curls, and squats, individuals can strengthen their muscles without putting excessive strain on their joints.

Water aerobics also promotes flexibility and range of motion. The water's natural resistance allows for a full range of motion in joints, enhancing flexibility. The water's buoyancy aids in stretching, making it easier to perform stretching exercises. As a result, water aerobics is an excellent option for individuals looking to improve their flexibility or recover from an injury.

Another health benefit of water aerobics is improved cardiovascular endurance. The consistent resistance from the water during exercise provides a great cardiovascular workout, increasing heart rate and strengthening the heart muscle. Regular water aerobics can help decrease the risk of heart disease, high blood pressure, and stroke.

Water aerobics is a highly effective exercise that offers numerous health and fitness benefits. The reduced impact on joints and bones, increased muscular strength and flexibility, and improved cardiovascular health make water aerobics a great choice for individuals of all ages and fitness levels. Incorporating water aerobics into a fitness routine not only provides an enjoyable way to stay active but also contributes significantly to overall health and well-being.

CAN I DO WATER AEROBICS IF I CAN'T SWIM?

Yes, you can do water aerobics even if you can't swim. Water aerobics is a low-impact exercise performed in waist or chest-deep water. The buoyancy of the water provides support, making it a safe and effective workout option for non-swimmers. You don't need to be able to swim or have any prior experience in the water to participate in water aerobics. It's a great way to improve cardiovascular fitness, strength, and flexibility while minimizing the risk of injury.

HOW OFTEN SHOULD I DO WATER AEROBICS?

The frequency of water aerobics largely depends on your fitness goals, physical condition, and schedule. As a general guideline, it is recommended to engage in water aerobics at least two to three times a week for beginners. More experienced individuals or those aiming for weight loss or improved cardiovascular health may benefit from doing it four to five times a week. Always consult with a fitness professional to determine the best frequency for your specific needs and capabilities.

2

GETTING STARTED WITH WATER AEROBICS

1. Choose the right location: Find a local community center or gym that offers water aerobics classes specifically tailored for seniors. These classes are usually designed to suit different fitness levels and abilities.

2. Get the right gear: Invest in proper swimwear and aqua shoes with good traction to prevent slipping. Aqua gloves or resistance paddles can be added for an extra challenge.

3. Warm-up and stretch: Just like any other exercise, water aerobics requires a proper warm-up routine before diving into the main workout. Start with gentle stretches to loosen up muscles.

4. Start slowly and progress gradually: As a beginner, it's important not to overexert yourself. Begin with basic movements, such as marching or walking in the water, and slowly increase the intensity and complexity of exercises as you become more comfortable.

5. Stay hydrated: Even though you are exercising in water, it's essential to stay hydrated. Bring a water

bottle with you and take sips during breaks.

6. Listen to your body: Pay attention to any signs of discomfort or pain. If you experience any unusual symptoms, stop exercising and consult your doctor or fitness instructor.

After, All that's left is to Grab your swimsuit, dive in, and enjoy the many benefits of water exercises

CHOOSING THE RIGHT POOL OR WATER AEROBICS CLASS

With the variety of classes available, it is essential for seniors to choose the right one that suits their specific needs and interests.

First and foremost, seniors should consider finding a class that caters to their level of fitness and ability. Some classes are specifically designed for beginners, while others may cater to more advanced participants. Seniors should start with a class that matches their current physical condition and gradually progress to more challenging classes as they become more comfortable in the water.

Another crucial aspect to look for when choosing a water aerobics or pool exercise class is the instructor's expertise. It is vital for seniors to ensure that the instructor is knowledgeable and experienced in working with older adults. A competent instructor will be able to modify exercises and provide adaptations for individuals with differing abilities or physical limitations.

Seniors should also consider the class schedule and location when making their decision. Opting for a class that fits into their routine and is conveniently located will increase the likelihood of attending regularly. Regular participation is crucial for reaping the full benefits of water exercise, such as improved cardiovascular health, muscle strength, and flexibility.

Furthermore, seniors should inquire about the class size and the availability of equipment. Smaller classes allow for more individual attention from the instructor and a safer and more personalized workout experience. Additionally, having access to appropriate equipment, such as flotation devices or resistance equipment, can enhance the effectiveness of the exercise program.

Lastly, seniors should consider the social aspect of the class. Participating in a group exercise class not only promotes physical well-being but also provides opportunities for social interaction and a sense of community. Seniors should choose a class that fosters a friendly and supportive atmosphere, enabling them to enjoy their exercise routine with like-minded individuals.

When choosing a pool or water aerobics class, seniors should consider their fitness level, the instructor's expertise, the schedule and location, class size and available equipment, and the social aspect. By taking these factors into account, seniors can select the right class that will suit their individual needs and preferences, ensuring a safe, enjoyable, and effective exercise experience.

SAFETY GUIDELINES FOR SENIORS IN THE WATER

As seniors age, staying active and maintaining good physical health become increasingly important. Engaging in water activities, like swimming or water aerobics, can provide numerous benefits for seniors. However, it is vital to follow safety guidelines to ensure a fun and accident-free experience in the water.

When swimming, seniors should never swim alone and should always have a buddy present, in case of any emergency. Moreover, it may be beneficial for them to learn basic water rescue techniques or CPR to be prepared for any potential incidents.

Wearing appropriate water safety gear such as life jackets or floatation devices can provide an extra layer of protection while in the water. These can be especially important for those with limited mobility or medical conditions.

Seniors should be aware of the risks associated with water, such as slippery surfaces and pool edges. It is crucial to take extra precautions when entering and exiting the water to prevent falls or injuries.

By following these safety guidelines, seniors can enjoy the benefits of water activities while minimizing the risk of accidents or injuries.

ESSENTIAL EQUIPMENT FOR WATER AEROBICS SESSIONS

Water aerobics is a fantastic exercise option for seniors due to its low impact nature. It can improve cardiovascular health, strengthen muscles, and enhance flexibility. To fully engage in water aerobics sessions, certain equipment is essential.

First and foremost, seniors should invest in a swimsuit designed for fitness activities in water. These suits offer good coverage and support, ensuring comfort and ease of movement. Additionally, water shoes or aqua socks can provide seniors with stability on slippery surfaces, protecting them from falls and injuries. These water shoes should have a non-slip sole for added safety.

A flotation belt or vest is another crucial piece of equipment for seniors in water aerobics. It offers buoyancy and support, allowing individuals to maintain an upright position and exercise with reduced impact on joints. Seniors should also consider using foam dumbbells or water noodles to add resistance to their workouts, enhancing muscle strength and endurance.

Lastly, a waterproof watch or timer can help seniors keep track of time and intensity during their sessions. This way, they can ensure they are exercising for an appropriate duration and intensity, avoiding overexertion.

Investing in the necessary equipment is a worthwhile investment for seniors engaged in water aerobics sessions. These items provide safety, comfort, and a more effective workout, enabling seniors to enjoy the numerous health benefits of this enjoyable exercise modality.

3

WATER AEROBICS EXERCISES FOR SENIORS

WARM-UP EXERCISES

Warm-up exercises are essential before any exercise routine as they increase blood flow, loosen muscles, and prepare the body for more strenuous activities. In water aerobics, warm-up exercises are specifically designed to target the major muscle groups while incorporating water resistance to provide additional challenges.

One common warm-up exercise in water aerobics is marching in place. This exercise helps mobilize the lower body and gets the heart rate up. Marching can be performed with high knees or low impact, depending on the individual's fitness level and range of motion.

Another beneficial warm-up exercise is the arm circle. This exercise targets the upper body and helps improve shoulder mobility and flexibility. By performing large, controlled circles with the arms, seniors can warm up and stretch out their shoulder muscles.

Stretching exercises such as toe-touches, side

lunges, and leg swings are also common warm-up exercises in water aerobics. These exercises improve flexibility and range of motion, preventing injuries and promoting better overall physical performance during the workout.

Warm-up exercises are essential to prepare the body for a safe and effective workout session. These exercises target the major muscle groups, increase blood flow, and improve flexibility. Engaging in warm-up exercises before water aerobics helps seniors prevent injuries, enhances overall physical well-being, and makes the workout experience more enjoyable.

ARM CIRCLES

Arm circles are a simple yet effective exercise that targets several upper body muscles. To perform arm circles, start by standing tall with your feet shoulder-width apart. Extend both arms straight out to your sides at shoulder level. Begin making small circular motions with your arms by moving them forward. Gradually increase the size of the circles to engage your shoulder, upper back, and chest muscles. Reverse the direction of the circles after a desired number of repetitions to target different muscle fibers. Arm circles can help improve shoulder mobility, strengthen the muscles around the shoulder joint, and enhance overall upper body strength and stability. Regular practice of arm circles can contribute to better posture and reduce the risk of shoulder-related injuries.

HIP ROTATIONS

Hip rotations are an excellent exercise for strengthening and mobilizing the hip joints. This simple movement involves rotating the hips in a circular motion, which helps improve flexibility, stability, and overall range of motion in the hips.

To perform hip rotations, stand with your feet hip-width apart and place your hands on your hips for support. Start by rotating your hips in a clockwise direction, making slow and controlled circles. As you become more comfortable with the movement, you can increase the size of the circles and the speed.

Hip rotations target the muscles of the hips, including the glutes, hip flexors, and hip abductors. By engaging these muscles, hip rotations help improve hip stability and alignment, reduce the risk of hip injuries, and enhance overall performance in activities such as running, jumping, and squatting.

Moreover, hip rotations can also relieve tension and tightness in the hip area, making them an excellent exercise for individuals who spend a lot of time sitting or have a sedentary lifestyle. Adding hip rotations to your regular exercise routine can help you maintain healthy hips and improve your overall functional movement.

TOE TOUCHES

Toe touches are a popular exercise that targets the core muscles and boosts flexibility. To perform this simple yet effective movement, start by standing tall with your feet hip-width apart. Engage your core muscles and reach your arms above your head. Keeping your back straight, hinge at your hips and simultaneously lift one leg straight up in front of you while reaching your opposite hand to touch your toes. Return to the starting position and repeat on the other side. Toe touches help improve balance, strengthen the abdominal muscles, and enhance hamstring flexibility. They can be modified to suit different fitness levels and can be easily incorporated into any workout routine.

CARDIOVASCULAR EXERCISES

Water aerobic cardiovascular exercises are a great way to improve cardiovascular fitness and overall health. These exercises involve performing various movements in the water, using the resistance of the water to increase the intensity of the workout.

Unlike traditional aerobic exercises, water aerobics is low-impact, making it suitable for people of all fitness levels and ages, including those with joint problems or injuries. The buoyancy of the water reduces the stress on the joints while providing resistance, resulting in a challenging workout without straining the body.

Some popular water aerobic cardiovascular exercises include water jogging, water walking, jumping jacks, and kicking movements. These exercises engage multiple muscle groups simultaneously, making them highly effective in increasing heart rate, burning calories, and improving cardiovascular endurance.

Furthermore, water aerobic cardiovascular exercises provide additional benefits such as improved balance, increased muscle strength, and enhanced flexibility. The water's buoyancy also helps to support the body, reducing the risk of injuries.

Whether you are a beginner or advanced fitness enthusiast, water aerobic cardiovascular exercises offer a fun and refreshing way to stay active and maintain a healthy heart. So why not dive in and give it a try?

WATER WALKING

Water walking, also known as aqua jogging or hydro-jogging, is a fantastic low-impact exercise that offers numerous benefits. It involves walking or jogging in a pool, typically waist-deep, to create resistance and buoyancy. This activity is perfect for people of all ages and fitness levels, especially seniors or those recovering from injuries or with joint problems.

Water walking offers many advantages. Firstly, it provides a full-body workout by engaging all major muscle groups, including the core, arms, and legs. The resistance from the water increases the intensity of the exercise, making it more effective for toning muscles and burning calories.

Additionally, water walking reduces the impact on joints and bones, making it a safe alternative to traditional walking or jogging. The buoyancy of the water supports your body, reducing the risk of injury while still providing a challenging cardiovascular workout. It is an excellent way to improve cardiovascular endurance and maintain overall fitness without straining your joints.

Water walking can also aid in rehabilitation and recovery from injuries. The water's buoyancy reduces weight-bearing, allowing for a gentle and controlled workout. It helps to rebuild strength and mobility without risking further damage.

Water walking is a highly beneficial exercise that promotes cardiovascular fitness, muscular strength, and joint health. Whether you are looking to lose weight, recover from an injury, or maintain overall fitness, water walking provides a low-impact, enjoyable, and effective workout option.

JOGGING IN PLACE

Jogging in place in water is an excellent exercise option for seniors who are looking to maintain their fitness levels or improve their overall health. This low-impact workout provides numerous benefits without putting excessive strain on joints and muscles.

Water jogging combines the cardiovascular benefits of jogging with the added resistance of water, resulting in a more efficient and effective workout. The buoyancy of water helps to support and cushion the body, reducing the risk of injury, making it a safe choice for older adults.

This exercise helps to improve strength, flexibility, and balance, which are key elements in maintaining a healthy lifestyle. By jogging in water, seniors can strengthen their core muscles, improve posture, and increase endurance. Additionally, the water's resistance helps to build muscle strength, leading to better mobility and reducing the risk of falls.

Another advantage of water jogging is its cooling effect, which minimizes the risk of overheating, especially for seniors who may be more susceptible to heat-related illnesses. Moreover, being in the water provides a sense of relaxation and reduces stress and anxiety.

Whether performed in a pool or a therapeutic tank, jogging in place in water is a low-impact, gentle exercise that seniors can enjoy and benefit from. It is an excellent option for maintaining physical fitness, improving overall health, and enhancing the quality of life for seniors.

KICKBOARDING

Kickboarding in water is an excellent form of exercise for seniors. It provides a low-impact workout that is easy on the joints while still improving cardiovascular health, muscular strength, and balance. This activity involves using a kickboard to kick and propel oneself through the water, providing resistance that works the leg muscles and helps improve overall strength.

For seniors, kickboarding in water offers a safe and enjoyable way to stay active and maintain a healthy lifestyle. The buoyancy of water reduces the risk of injury, making it an ideal exercise for those with arthritis or joint pain. It also helps improve flexibility and range of motion, enhancing the seniors' overall physical condition.

Additionally, kickboarding in water has many mental health benefits. Being in water has a calming effect on the mind, reducing stress levels and promoting relaxation. It can also serve as a social activity, allowing seniors to connect with others and make new friends. This social interaction is crucial for combating loneliness and depression, issues that can affect seniors' mental well-being.

Kickboarding in water is an excellent exercise option for seniors. It helps improve physical fitness, offers a low-impact workout, and provides mental health benefits. By incorporating kickboarding into their routine, seniors can maintain a healthy and active lifestyle while enjoying the many advantages that water-based exercise provides.

STRENGTH AND RESISTANCE EXERCISES

Strength and resistance exercises in water have proven to be highly beneficial for seniors. Water offers a low-impact environment that minimizes stress on joints, making it ideal for older adults who have arthritis or other mobility issues. These exercises not only improve strength but also enhance flexibility and balance.

Water provides resistance in all directions, resulting in a full-body workout. Seniors can perform various exercises such as water walking or jogging, leg lifts, arm curls, and torso twists, all of which help to build muscle tone and improve cardiovascular fitness. The resistance of the water forces the muscles to work harder than they would on land, leading to improved strength and endurance.

Water exercises promote joint mobility and reduce pain. The buoyancy of water supports the body, reducing the risk of falls and injuries, enabling seniors to perform exercises they may not be able to do on land. Water also offers natural resistance and helps to decrease swelling, allowing seniors to move their joints more easily and effectively.

Strength and resistance exercises in water are a perfect choice for seniors. They provide numerous physical benefits, including increased muscle strength, improved flexibility, enhanced balance, and reduced joint pain. Water exercises are enjoyable, safe, and effective, making them an excellent fitness option for older adults aiming to maintain their overall health and wellbeing.

LEG LIFTS

Leg lifts in water are a fantastic exercise option for seniors. As we age, our joints and muscles can become less flexible and more prone to injury. Water-based exercises, such as leg lifts, provide a low-impact way of keeping the body active and improving overall strength.

Water provides natural resistance, making leg lifts more challenging and effective than if performed on land. This resistance helps to strengthen the muscles in the legs, including the quadriceps, hamstrings, and glutes. These muscle groups are crucial for maintaining balance and stability, which are essential for older adults.

The buoyancy of water also reduces the impact on joints, making it ideal for seniors who experience joint pain or stiffness. Leg lifts in water are gentle on the knees and hips, making it a safe choice for individuals with arthritis or other orthopedic conditions.

Exercising in water can improve cardiovascular health and increase range of motion, helping seniors maintain their independence and mobility. Additionally, water-based exercises have been shown to alleviate symptoms of chronic conditions such as fibromyalgia and osteoporosis.

Leg lifts in water offer numerous benefits for seniors, including increased strength, improved balance, reduced joint impact, and improved overall well-being. It is a safe and enjoyable way for seniors to stay active and maintain a high quality of life.

ARM CURLS

Water exercises are ideal for seniors as they offer a low-impact way to maintain strength and improve overall fitness. One specific exercise that can be highly beneficial for seniors is arm curls in water.

Arm curls in water involve standing in a pool or

another body of water with water at chest level. Seniors can then use water dumbbells or simply their own body resistance to perform bicep curls. This exercise primarily targets the biceps but also engages the muscles in the forearms and shoulders.

Engaging in arm curls in water offers several advantages for seniors. Firstly, the buoyancy of water reduces the impact on joints, making it easier to perform the exercise without undue strain or risk of injury. Additionally, the water provides resistance throughout the range of motion, which helps strengthen and tone the arm muscles more effectively than performing arm curls on land.

Moreover, water exercises are particularly beneficial for seniors with arthritis or other joint conditions, as the water's buoyancy and warmth can help alleviate pain and stiffness.

Arm curls in water offer seniors a safe and effective way to build arm strength, improve muscle tone, and promote overall fitness. This low-impact exercise can be easily incorporated into water fitness routines, making it a valuable addition to senior exercise programs.

WATER DUMBBELL EXERCISES

Water dumbbell exercises for seniors are an excellent way to stay active and maintain strength and flexibility. As we age, it becomes crucial to focus on exercises that are low-impact and gentle on the joints, and water dumbbell exercises perfectly fit the bill.

Water offers natural resistance that helps to tone muscles without putting excessive stress on the body. Seniors can comfortably perform various exercises such as bicep curls, tricep extensions, lateral raises, and front arm raises using water dumbbells. These exercises help to strengthen the upper body, including the arms, shoulders, and chest, improving overall functionality and reducing the risk of injury.

To perform bicep curls, tricep extensions, lateral raises, and front arm raises using water dumbbells, follow these steps:

1. Start by standing in an upright position with your feet shoulder-width apart. Hold a water dumbbell in each hand, ensuring a firm grip on the handles.

2. Bicep Curls:

Keep your upper arms stationary and close to your

body throughout the exercise.

Bend your elbows and raise the dumbbells towards your shoulders.

Slowly lower the dumbbells back to the starting position. Repeat for the desired number of repetitions.

3. Tricep Extensions:

Raise both dumbbells above your head, with your arms fully extended.

Bend your elbows, slowly lowering the dumbbells behind your head.

Extend your arms back up, returning to the starting position. Repeat for the desired number of repetitions.

4. Lateral Raises:

Hold the dumbbells by your sides, palms facing inward.

Keeping your arms straight, lift both dumbbells out to the sides until they reach shoulder height.

Slowly lower the dumbbells back to the starting position. Repeat for the desired number of repetitions.

5. Front Arm Raises:

Hold the dumbbells in front of your thighs, palms facing your body.

With your arms straight, lift both dumbbells forward until they reach shoulder height.

Slowly lower the dumbbells back to the starting position. Repeat for the desired number of repetitions.

Remember to start with lighter weights and gradually increase the resistance as you gain strength. It is crucial to maintain proper form and control throughout each exercise to maximize their effectiveness and prevent injury.

Water dumbbell exercises improve cardiovascular endurance without causing strain on the heart. The buoyancy of water supports the body, making it an ideal exercise medium for seniors who may have balance issues or frailty concerns.

Including water dumbbell exercises in a regular exercise routine can also aid in weight management, improving posture, and relieving joint pain and stiffness.

Water dumbbell exercises offer a safe and effective way for seniors to enhance their physical fitness. These exercises promote strength, flexibility, cardiovascular endurance, and overall well-being in a gentle and enjoyable manner.

KNEE EXCERCISES

Water exercises are a fantastic way for seniors to engage in low-impact workouts that are gentle on their joints, and knee exercises in particular can help improve strength, flexibility, and overall function.

Water provides a supportive environment that reduces pressure on the knees while still providing resistance for the muscles. Senior citizens can perform a variety of knee exercises in water, such as knee raises, leg extensions, and squats. These exercises help target the muscles surrounding the knee joint and promote stability.

Water exercises have gained popularity in recent years due to the numerous benefits they offer. Knee raises, leg extensions, and squats in water are three effective exercises that can help improve strength, flexibility, and cardiovascular fitness while minimizing the risk of injury.

1. Knee Raises: Knee raises in water are a great way to target the abdominal muscles, hip flexors, and quadriceps. Start by standing in chest-deep water with your feet shoulder-width apart. Hold onto the pool's edge for balance if needed. Lift one knee towards your chest while keeping your back straight. Lower the leg back down and repeat on the other side. Aim for 10-15 repetitions per leg. You can also increase the intensity by adding ankle weights or using a kickboard.

2. Leg Extensions: Leg extensions in water primarily target the quadriceps, hamstrings, and glutes. Begin by standing in waist-deep water with your legs together. Hold onto the pool's edge for stability if required. Slowly extend one leg in front of you, pointing your toes towards the surface of the water. Flex your foot as you return the leg back to the starting position. Repeat with the other leg. Aim for 10-15 repetitions per leg. You can modify this exercise by using resistance bands around your ankles or incorporating ankle weights.

3. Squats: Squats in water help strengthen the glutes, quadriceps, hamstrings, and core muscles. Stand with your feet shoulder-width apart in chest-deep water. Extend your arms in front of you for balance. Keeping your back straight, lower yourself

into a squat position by bending your knees and sitting back like you're sitting on an imaginary chair. Ensure your knees do not go past your toes. Return to the starting position and repeat the movement for 10-15 repetitions. To increase the difficulty, try doing squats on one leg or using water dumbbells for resistance.

Performing knee raises, leg extensions, and squats in water provides a low-impact workout that is gentle on the joints while still effectively improving muscle strength and endurance. Additionally, the resistance offered by the water helps tone and challenge the muscles. These exercises can be beneficial for individuals of all fitness levels, making them a great choice for rehabilitation, weight loss, or simply adding variety to your workout routine. Remember to consult with a healthcare professional before starting any new exercise program, especially if you have any pre-existing conditions or injuries.

Additionally, water provides natural resistance, making movements more challenging and effective without putting excessive strain on the knees. The buoyancy of water also allows seniors to perform exercises that may be difficult on land due to balance issues or joint discomfort.

Water exercises for the knees also offer numerous other benefits for seniors, including increased circulation, improved cardiovascular health, and enhanced balance and coordination. Regular participation in water exercises can help seniors maintain a healthy weight, reduce the risk of falls, and manage conditions such as arthritis and osteoporosis.

Overall, knee exercises in water offer a safe and effective way for seniors to maintain their mobility, strengthen their knees, and improve their overall fitness.

ARTHRITIS EXERCISES

Arthritis exercises in water prove to be highly beneficial for seniors who suffer from joint pain and stiffness. Water provides a supportive and low-impact environment, reducing the strain on joints and facilitating better mobility.

Water exercises for seniors with arthritis focus on improving range of motion, flexibility, and strength. Water buoyancy helps to reduce the load on joints, allowing you to move more freely without exacerbating pain. Gentle movements like water walking, water aerobics, and basic water stretches target various muscle groups without putting excessive stress on joints. The resistance offered by water also helps in building strength over time.

Furthermore, working out in water improves circulation and reduces inflammation, providing relief to arthritic joints. Warm water, in particular, can help soothe aching joints and provide additional comfort. Regular water exercises can enhance joint flexibility, maintain muscle tone, and improve overall function.

Importantly, water exercises are suitable for individuals with all levels of fitness, making them an ideal choice for seniors with arthritis. It is always recommended to consult with a healthcare professional or a physical therapist before starting any exercise program, to ensure appropriate exercises are chosen that match individual capabilities and needs.

HIP EXERCISES

Hip exercises in water can be highly beneficial for seniors as they provide a low-impact and gentle way to improve hip mobility and muscle strength. Water helps to reduce the stress on joints, making it an ideal environment for seniors with conditions such as arthritis or those recovering from hip surgery.

One effective exercise is water marching, which involves lifting each knee up towards the chest alternately while standing in waist-deep water. This exercise helps to strengthen the hip flexor muscles and improve balance and coordination. Another exercise is leg swings, which can be performed by standing near the pool side and swinging one leg forward and backward while holding on for support. This exercise targets the hip abductor and adductor muscles.

Water-based exercises like squats or hip raises are also helpful in strengthening the hip muscles. Wearing a flotation belt or using a pool noodle for support can assist seniors in maintaining balance during these exercises. To do hip raises in water, start by standing in waist-deep water. Place your hands on the poolside or floatation device for stability. Lift one leg at a time, bending at the knee and raising it towards your chest. Hold for a few seconds, then lower it back down. Repeat with the other leg. Additionally, walking in water on tiptoes or performing hip circles can help improve range of motion and flexibility in the hip joints.

Engaging in a regular water-based exercise routine not only improves hip strength and flexibility but also promotes cardiovascular fitness and helps maintain a healthy weight. However, seniors should always consult with a healthcare professional or a physical therapist before starting any new exercise program.

SHOULDER EXERCISES

Shoulder exercises in water can be extremely beneficial for seniors in maintaining and improving their shoulder strength, flexibility, and range of motion. As we age, our shoulders tend to weaken, leading to reduced mobility and increased risk of injury. However, exercising in water provides a low-impact environment that reduces strain on joints and minimizes the risk of falls or accidents.

By performing exercises such as shoulder rotations, arm raises, and gentle stretches in water, seniors can improve their overall shoulder mobility and flexibility, increasing their ability to perform daily activities with ease.

Shoulder Rotations:

1. Stand with your feet shoulder-width apart and your hands resting on your hips.

2. Slowly rotate your shoulders forward in a circular motion, starting with small circles and gradually increasing the size.

3. After completing several rotations forward, switch to rotating your shoulders backward in a circular motion.

4. Repeat the forward and backward rotations, adjusting the speed and size of the circles based on your comfort level.

Arm Raises:

5. Stand with your feet shoulder-width apart, keeping your core engaged.

6. Begin by raising one arm straight in front of you, bringing it up until it is parallel to the water surface.

7. Slowly lower the arm back down and repeat with the other arm.

8. Alternate raising and lowering your arms in front of you, focusing on proper form and control.

GENTLE STRETCHES:

1. Extend your arms out to the sides, parallel to the water surface.

2. Gently reach your arms backward until you feel a comfortable stretch in your chest and shoulders. Hold this position for 10-15 seconds.

3. Bring your arms back to the starting position and then slowly reach your arms forward until you feel a gentle stretch in your upper back and shoulders. Hold for 10-15 seconds.

4. Repeat these stretches, alternating between the stretch to the back and front, focusing on maintaining proper form and avoiding any discomfort.

5. To stretch your neck, slowly tilt your head to the left, bringing your left ear closer to your left shoulder. Hold for 10-15 seconds before repeating on the right side.

6. Continue with other gentle stretches as desired, such as arm crosses, full-body stretches, or calf stretches while leaning against a pool wall.

Listen to your body, take it at your own pace, and stop any exercise if you feel pain or discomfort.

Water exercises also relieve joint pain and stiffness, making it feasible for seniors with arthritis or other conditions to engage in effective shoulder workouts. Regular water exercises can help alleviate pain, reduce inflammation, and increase blood flow, contributing to better overall joint health. Additionally, exercising in water enhances balance and stability, reducing the likelihood of falls and fractures.

Shoulder exercises in water serve as a safe and effective way for seniors to maintain and enhance their shoulder strength and flexibility, enabling them to lead active and independent lifestyles. However, it is recommended to consult with a healthcare professional or a certified aquatic therapist before starting any exercise regimen.

BACK AND WAIST EXERCISES

Water exercises are highly beneficial for seniors, particularly when it comes to strengthening their back and waist muscles. Exercising in water provides a low-impact environment that reduces strain on joints, making it an ideal option for elderly individuals with limited mobility or joint pain.

One of the most effective back exercises for seniors in water is the water walking exercise. To perform this exercise, seniors can walk forward, backward, or sideways in waist-deep water, focusing on maintaining proper posture and engaging core muscles. The resistance of the water helps engage and strengthen the muscles in the back and waist, enhancing flexibility and stability.

Another effective exercise is the water twist. Seniors can stand in chest-deep water and, using their core muscles, twist their hips from side to side. This exercise helps improve posture, strengthen the waist, and increase flexibility.

Senior aquatic classes led by trained instructors can provide a structured and safe environment for seniors to engage in water back and waist exercises.

Water exercises offer seniors a safe and effective way to strengthen their back and waist muscles. Incorporating these exercises into a regular exercise routine can contribute to improved mobility, flexibility, and overall well-being in seniors.

FLEXIBILITY AND STRETCHING EXERCISES

Flexibility and stretching exercises in water offer incredible benefits for seniors. The buoyancy of water reduces the impact on joints, making it ideal for individuals with arthritis or joint pain. Gentle movements in water strengthen muscles, improve balance, and increase range of motion. These exercises can be performed in shallow water or with the support of flotation devices. Water provides natural resistance that helps seniors build muscle strength without straining their muscles or causing injuries. Moreover, water-based workouts can enhance cardiovascular health, reduce stress, and improve overall well-being. Incorporating a regular routine of flexibility and stretching exercises in water can promote joint health, maintain flexibility, and increase mobility in seniors.

SIDE STRETCHES

Side stretches in water are an excellent form of exercise for seniors, providing gentle yet effective movements to improve flexibility and reduce muscle stiffness. The buoyancy of water reduces the strain on joints, making it a low-impact workout that is safe for aging bodies. This exercise specifically targets the muscles on the sides of the body, including the obliques and intercostal muscles. By extending one arm overhead and reaching towards the opposite direction, seniors can lengthen and strengthen these muscles. Regular practice of side stretches in water can enhance posture, increase range of motion, and alleviate back pain, promoting overall wellness for seniors.

CHEST OPENER

The chest opener exercise in water is a fantastic option for those looking to improve their upper body strength and flexibility.

To perform the chest opener, seniors can simply stand in water, with the water level reaching their chest. They can then extend their arms out to the sides and slowly bring them forward, crossing them in front of their body, and then return to the starting position. This exercise effectively stretches and strengthens the chest, shoulders, and upper back muscles.

The water's buoyancy helps reduce stress on the joints, making it easier for seniors to perform the movement. Additionally, the resistance offered by the water enhances muscle engagement, contributing to improved strength and flexibility. The chest opener in water is an excellent choice for seniors to maintain and enhance their overall upper body health.

CALF STRETCHES

Calf stretches in water can be an excellent exercise for seniors. Calf stretches target the muscles in the lower leg, promoting flexibility, range of motion, and circulation. To perform calf stretches in water, stand in waist-deep water, facing the poolside.

Place your hands on the pool edge for support. Step one foot forward, keeping the other leg straight. Lean forward and feel the stretch in your back calf. Hold for 15-30 seconds and repeat with the other leg.. This exercise helps to alleviate stiffness, cramps, and pain in the lower leg, which is a common concern for older adults. Additionally, calf stretches in water provide a refreshing and enjoyable way for seniors to keep their legs limber and maintain overall mobility.

4

ADVANCED WATER AEROBICS TECHNIQUES FOR SENIORS

Advanced water aerobics techniques for seniors can offer numerous benefits, including improved cardiovascular health, muscle strength, and flexibility. To enhance their workout, seniors can incorporate these advanced techniques into their water aerobics routine.

One technique is deep water running, where seniors strap on a flotation belt and run in the deeper end of the pool without touching the bottom. This helps to increase their heart rate and engage the muscles of the lower body. Another technique is water resistance training, which involves using handheld water weights or resistance bands to perform various exercises such as bicep curls, shoulder presses, and leg extensions. This helps to build muscle strength and tone.

You can also benefit from using pool noodles or aqua dumbbells for additional resistance while performing exercises like squats or lunges in the shallow end of the pool. This helps to target the legs, glutes, and core muscles. Additionally, seniors can try water jogging or kickboxing exercises, which involve high-intensity movements that challenge their balance and help improve their cardiovascular fitness.

Proper form and technique are crucial to avoid strain or injury. By incorporating these advanced techniques into their water aerobics routine, seniors can maximize the benefits of their workouts and enjoy improved health and wellbeing.

DEEP WATER EXERCISES

Deep water exercises can be incredibly beneficial for seniors. Working out in deep water offers a low-impact, gentle approach to exercising. Not only does water buoyancy support the body, reducing strain on joints, but it also provides resistance, helping to build muscle strength.

Senior water exercises can include a variety of movements, such as water walking, jogging, or cycling. The unique properties of water create an environment where seniors can safely engage in aerobic activities, improving cardiovascular health and endurance. Additionally, water-based exercises promote better balance and stability, reducing the risk of falls.

Moreover, deep water exercises offer a reprieve from gravity, allowing seniors to move freely, stretching muscles and improving flexibility. From simple arm and leg movements to more complex exercises like water aerobics or tai chi, seniors can engage in a range of activities that are both enjoyable and beneficial for their overall well-being.

Tai Chi is an ancient Chinese practice that combines gentle, flowing movements with deep breathing and meditation. It has been widely recognized as a beneficial exercise for seniors due to its low-impact nature. One variation of Tai Chi, known as "Water Exercises," focuses on slow, fluid movements that mimic the flow of water.

Water exercises in Tai Chi offer numerous benefits for seniors. Firstly, they improve strength, flexibility, and balance, which are crucial for preventing falls and maintaining overall fitness. The slow, controlled movements also promote relaxation, reduce stress, and improve mental clarity, making it an ideal exercise for seniors coping with anxiety or cognitive decline.

Additionally, water exercises are gentle on the

joints, making them suitable for individuals with arthritis or other joint-related issues. The water provides resistance, which helps build muscle strength without putting excessive strain on the body. Moreover, the buoyancy of water reduces impact and increases support, which can alleviate joint pain and make exercising more comfortable.

Tai Chi Water Exercises are an ideal option for seniors seeking a low-impact, holistic exercise routine. The combination of fluid movements, deep breathing, and meditation provides physical, mental, and emotional benefits. Whether practiced in a pool or on dry land, this form of Tai Chi is a gentle yet effective exercise that can enhance the overall well-being of older adults.

Doing Tai Chi in water can provide a unique and invigorating experience, combining the fluidity of the movements with the resistance of water. To start, find a shallow and calm body of water. Stand in the water up to your waist, ensuring stability. Begin with gentle stretching, focusing on maintaining good posture and alignment. Slowly transition into the Tai Chi form while adjusting to the resistance of the water. Keep the movements slow and controlled, allowing the water to support and challenge your body simultaneously.

Emphasize deep and relaxed breathing throughout the practice. The water will add an extra element of balance and fluidity, creating a beautiful and calming Tai Chi experience.

Ultimately, deep water exercises can be a fun, safe, and effective way for seniors to stay active and maintain a healthy lifestyle.

WATER RESISTANCE EQUIPMENT

Water resistance equipment refers to specially designed tools and gear that allow individuals to workout and exercise in water. It is particularly popular in aquatic fitness classes and rehabilitation programs. These equipment items are designed to provide resistance against the natural resistance of water, intensifying the workout while minimizing the risk of injury.

Water resistance equipment includes a wide range of products such as buoyancy belts, resistance gloves, water dumbbells, resistance bands, and aqua bikes. Buoyancy belts are commonly used to provide support and floatability during water workouts, enabling users to focus on specific movements and target muscle groups with ease. Resistance gloves and water dumbbells add an extra layer of resistance against the water, enhancing the intensity of exercises like arm curls and punches.

The benefits of using water resistance equipment are numerous. Water-based workouts are gentle on the joints and offer an excellent way to improve cardiovascular fitness, muscular strength, and overall endurance. Furthermore, exercising in water also helps to improve balance, coordination, and flexibility. The resistance provided by the equipment adds a challenging element, making it ideal for individuals looking for varied and effective workouts.

Whether used for rehabilitation purposes, aquatic fitness classes, or simply as a fun way to exercise, water resistance equipment offers a unique and effective way to stay active in the water. Its increasing popularity is a testament to its effectiveness and versatility.

INTERVAL TRAINING IN THE WATER

Interval training in the water is a highly effective and popular form of exercise that combines cardiovascular conditioning with strength training. It involves alternating periods of high-intensity exercises with lower-intensity recovery periods. This type of training can be done in various water environments, such as swimming pools or the open sea, making it accessible to people of all fitness levels.

One of the advantages of interval training in the water is that it provides a low-impact workout, reducing the stress on joints, muscles, and bones. The buoyancy of water also helps to support body weight, making it an ideal exercise for individuals with injuries or those who are overweight.

Interval training in the water engages multiple muscle groups simultaneously due to the resistance provided by water. This results in a more efficient and intense workout, as compared to traditional land-based exercises. Additionally, water acts as a natural resistance, increasing the effort required during the workout and thereby aiding in burning more calories.

Interval training in the water can be customized to suit individual needs and fitness levels. It can be as simple as alternating between fast and slow swimming or involve using equipment like water weights or resistance bands. Regardless of the intensity or complexity, interval training in the water offers a fun and enjoyable way to improve cardiovascular endurance, strength, and overall fitness.

5

TIPS FOR SUCCESS IN WATER AEROBICS

Water aerobics is a fun and effective way to stay fit and healthy.

It's essential to choose the right equipment. Invest in a proper swimsuit that provides flexibility and support. A water aerobics belt or floatation device like a noodle can help you stay afloat and support your movements.

Find a qualified instructor or join a class. Their expertise will guide you through the exercises and ensure you are doing them correctly, optimizing the benefits and preventing injuries.

Setting realistic goals and tracking your progress is crucial. Whether it's increasing the intensity or duration of your workouts, keeping a journal will motivate and inspire you.

Make it enjoyable by varying your routines, interacting with fellow participants, and keeping a positive mindset. Remember, consistency is key, and by following these tips, you'll be on your way to achieving success in water aerobics.

STAYING HYDRATED

Staying hydrated during water aerobics is vital for maintaining optimal performance and overall health. As water activities can cause excessive sweating, it is necessary to replenish the fluids lost to prevent dehydration. Drinking enough water before, during, and after the workout is essential. A good rule of thumb is to aim for at least 8 ounces of water every 20 minutes of exercise. It is also important to listen to your body and drink when thirsty. Electrolyte-rich beverages, like sports drinks, can also help replace minerals lost through sweat. Hydration, combined with proper technique and regular breaks, ensures a safe and effective water aerobics session.

SETTING GOALS AND TRACKING PROGRESS

Setting goals and tracking progress in water aerobics is crucial for achieving desired outcomes and maintaining motivation. When starting a water aerobics routine, it is important to set specific and achievable goals. These goals can range from improving overall fitness and strength to specific targets like completing a certain number of laps or mastering a particular exercise. By setting goals, individuals can have a clear vision of what they want to accomplish and work towards it.

Tracking progress is equally essential as it helps monitor the results and make necessary adjustments. This can be done by measuring metrics such as heart rate, duration of workout, or distance covered. Regularly assessing progress enables individuals to identify areas of improvement, celebrate milestones, and stay accountable. Moreover, keeping a record of progress can inspire and maintain motivation, as it showcases the positive changes achieved over time.

In water aerobics, setting goals that are challenging yet attainable and tracking progress consistently are key to staying focused, pushing boundaries, and ultimately achieving desired fitness levels and maximum health benefits.

MAKING WATER AEROBICS A SOCIAL ACTIVITY

Water aerobics is a fun and invigorating way to stay fit, and adding a social aspect to it makes the experience even more enjoyable. By turning water aerobics into a social activity, participants can bond with others while exercising. This can be achieved by organizing group classes, encouraging conversations during breaks, and incorporating team-based exercises. Not only does this create a supportive and motivating environment, but it also helps individuals build friendships and form a sense of community. Making water aerobics a social activity ensures that seniors have a blast while working towards their fitness goals.

CONCLUSION

Water aerobics for seniors is an excellent option for older adults to stay active and maintain a healthy lifestyle. It offers numerous physical and mental benefits that cater specifically to their needs and capabilities.

Firstly, water aerobics is a low-impact exercise that reduces strain on joints, making it a safe and effective option for seniors. The buoyancy of water helps to support the body, alleviating pressure on the bones and muscles. This makes it an ideal form of exercise for those with arthritis, back pain, or balance issues. The decreased risk of injury allows seniors to engage in a regular fitness routine without fear.

Secondly, water aerobics offers a full-body workout that helps seniors improve their cardiovascular health, strength, and flexibility. The resistance provided by water increases muscle strength, leading to improved mobility and reduced risk of falls. The range of motion exercises in water help maintain joint flexibility and prevent stiffness. Additionally, the water pressure on the body aids in the circulation of blood, thus improving cardiovascular health and reducing the risk of chronic diseases, such as heart disease and diabetes, which are common among seniors.

Moreover, water aerobics provides a supportive and social environment for seniors to be active. Participating in group classes fosters a sense of community and camaraderie among participants. Seniors can make friends, share experiences, and motivate each other to maintain a healthy lifestyle. The social aspect of water aerobics offers mental and emotional well-being benefits, reducing stress, anxiety, and loneliness.

Overall, water aerobics for seniors is a fantastic way to promote overall wellness. It allows older adults to stay physically fit, maintain joint health, enhance cardiovascular function, and improve mental well-being. The low-impact nature of this exercise ensures safety, regardless of age or fitness level. The supportive and social environment encourages social interaction, making it an enjoyable and fulfilling experience for seniors. Therefore, water aerobics should be encouraged and promoted as a beneficial form of exercise for seniors to age gracefully and maintain their quality of life.

www.ingramcontent.com/pod-product-compliance
Lightning Source LLC
Chambersburg PA
CBHW050855260726
48660CB00006B/2645